Western Reiki Energy Medicine
The Healing Plan of Common Cold for Reiki Therapist

Reiki Protocol Card series #1 - Common Cold

by Dr.Jennifer Chou

Copyright @ 2018

Content

A Brief Anatomical Drawing

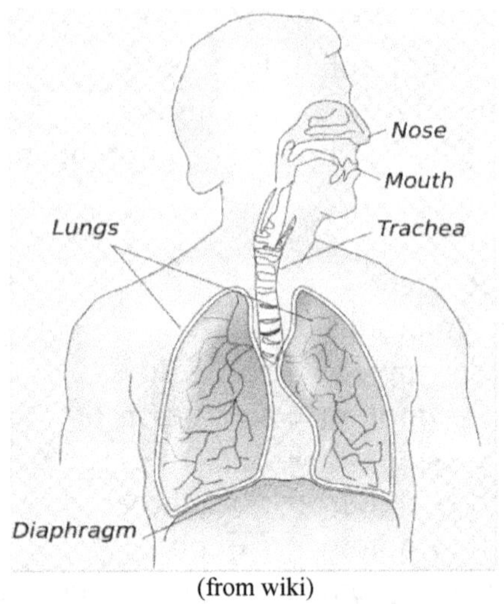

(from wiki)

Principles of medical science

Flu:

Of four types of influenza viruses that affect people, influenza A and B viruses are the ones that cause seasonal epidemics. Influenza, or the flu, and common colds have common symptoms, such as mucus congestion, sore throat, headaches, chest discomfort. High fever (above 103°F), body aches in the back, arms and legs, chills and sweats, nausea, weakness, and fatigue are common symptoms of the flu. Those with the flu are less likely to experience a runny nose than those with the common cold.

The flu usually lasts about 10 days, however complications can occur in those with immature or compromised immune systems. Pneumonia, bronchitis, sinus infections and ear infections are examples of flu-related complications. The flu also can make chronic health problems, such as asthma, heart disease, and lung disease, worse.

Common cold:

More than 200 virus strains can cause the common cold. Cold symptoms can begin in the first 10 to 12 hours after exposure, and the peak of symptoms is typically 36-72 hours after exposure. Symptoms of a common cold include a stuffy or runny nose, sore or scratchy throat, cough, and mild general symptoms like headache, low fever (up to 102°F), chilliness, and not feeling well in general. Colds rarely cause a fever or headaches. Colds last on average for one week. Mild colds may last only 2 or 3 days while severe colds may last for up to 2 weeks Adults average 2 to 3 colds per year.

This healing plan is designed for common cold. Flu symptoms such as fever, headache or systemic soreness may also be present in common cold patients although the percentage of such incidence is low.

Scan/Estimate

1. Each individual may present other health issues; thus, try not to be confused.

2. Manifestation of each individual differs at different stage of disease course.

3. Feel the scannable areas with hands: neck, back of head, forehead, eyes, mouth and nose, throat, chest and lung. Area(s) of soreness or headache.

4. In some individual cases, abnormal energy mass can be scanned at the intestine and stomach area or the heart and lung area.

Techniques

Apply both tonifying and reducing methods;

Tonifying method
Reducing method
Cleansing method
Balancing method
Infiltrating method

Meditation

Right brain healer: Countdown from 1 to 100, subtract 2 each time.

Left brain healer: Countdown from 100 to 1, subtract 2 each time.
Put yourself into alpha brain wave

Instruction of Reiki Healing Protocol
(Hand placements and techniques)

1. The healer should stick to the basic prescription regardless of the accompanied symptoms.

2. Accompanied symptoms
Except for the basic prescription for the chief complaint, any hand placement of the accompanied symptoms can be applied repeatedly.

3. Timing (min.)Healing time is counted by minute.
4. Techniques

Treatment Course Prescription Outline

(Hand placements and techniques)
1. Basic prescription 20'
2. Each accompanied symptom 10'
3. Ending: balance and grounding 5~10'
4. Combine: nutrition and nursing.
5. Attention, intention.

Reiki Healing Protocol

The treatment course is designed for different stages of disease,

1. At the initial stage of common cold, heal once a day for 1-3 days.

2. At the middle stage of common cold, heal once every 2 days, approximately twice in 4 days.

3. For prolonged common cold, medical treatment can be included to facilitate the improvement.

Basic Protocol Chief complaint
- Common cold

Hand Placements

Main Hand Placements

1. Hand Placements: Lung area on the back => 2. neck =>
3. back of head => 4. lung area of the chest
2. Timing: 20' (min)
3. Techniques: first tonifying and then infiltrating method
in every hand placement

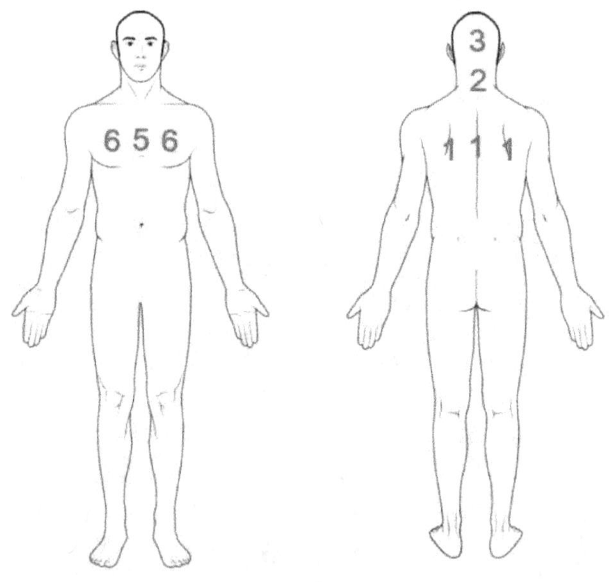

Accompanied symptom

Hand placements vary depending on the accompanied symptoms. In case of more than one accompanied symptom, hand placements can be repeated.

Accompanied symptom + feel cold

1. Hand placements: Back => neck => back of head
2. Timing: 10'

3. Techniques: tonifying + balancing method

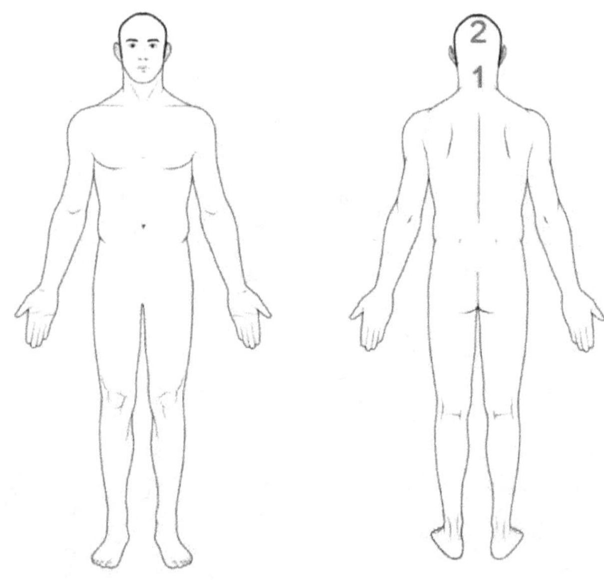

Accompanied symptom + feel warm

1. Hand placements: Back => neck => back of head
2. Timing: 10'
3. Techniques: Reducing + balancing method

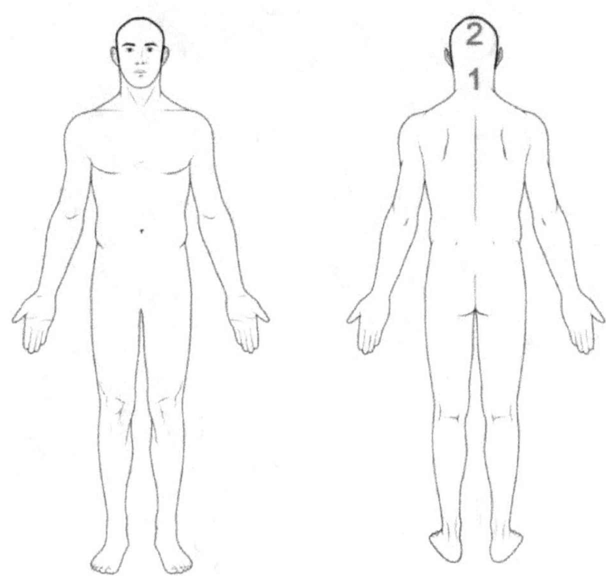

Accompanied symptom + feel tired

1. Hand placements: Overhead => heart and chest area => upper abdomen
2. Timing: 10'

3. Techniques: tonifying + balancing method

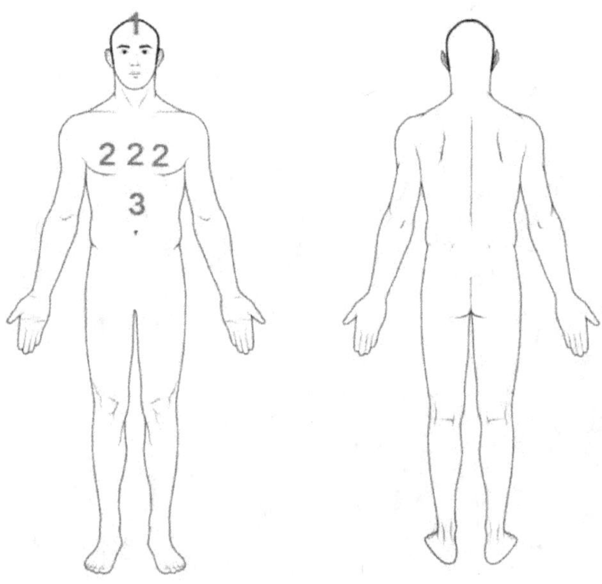

Accompanied symptom + Sneezing. Runny nose

1. Hand placements: Forehead => eyes => nose => paranasal sinus
2. Timing: 10'
3. Techniques: Cleansing + reducing infiltrating methods

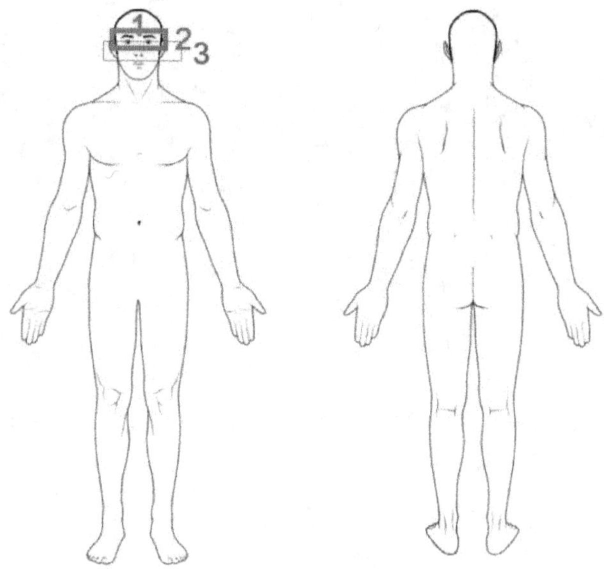

Accompanied symptom + Sore throat

1. Hand placements: Throat => stomach => intestine
2. Timing: 10'
3. Techniques: Cleansing + reducing infiltrating methods

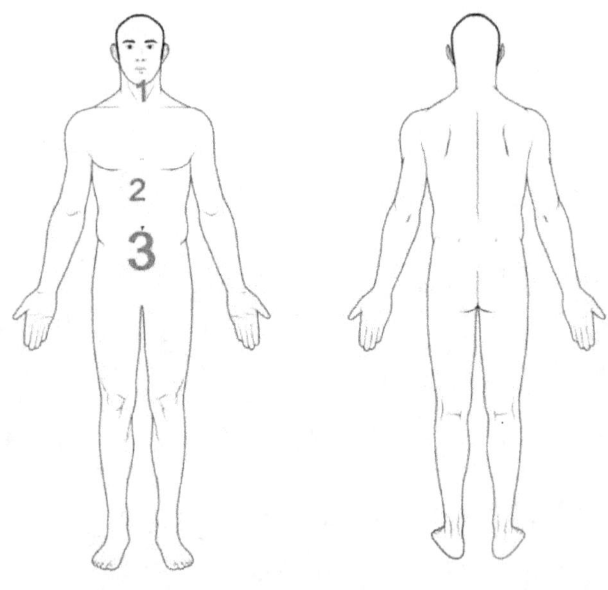

Accompanied symptom + Cough

1. Hand placements: Nose => mouth => throat=> lung
2. Timing: 10'
3. Techniques: Cleansing + reducing + tonifying,
infiltrating methods

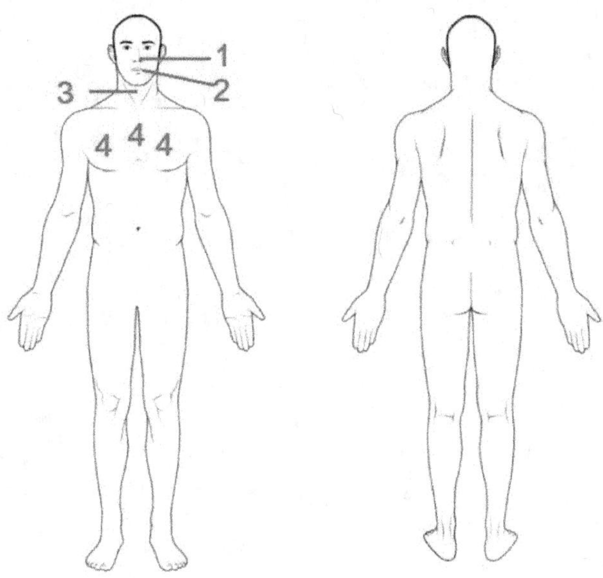

Accompanied symptom + Congestion problem

1. Hand placements: Stomach => small intestine => large intestine => knees
2. Timing: 10'
3. Techniques: Cleansing + reducing in3filtrating methods
Note: keep your belly warm

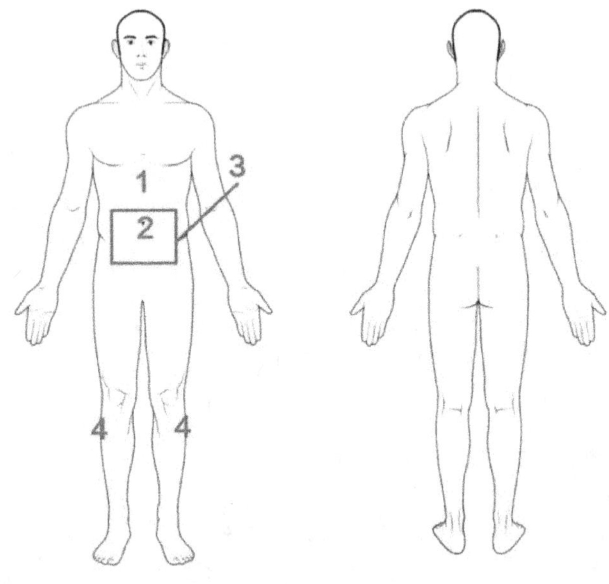

Accompanied symptom + body aches or a mild headache

1. Hand placements: Overhead => lateral head => chest and hypochondrium => stomach area
2. Timing: 10'
3. Techniques: Cleansing + reducing infiltrating methods

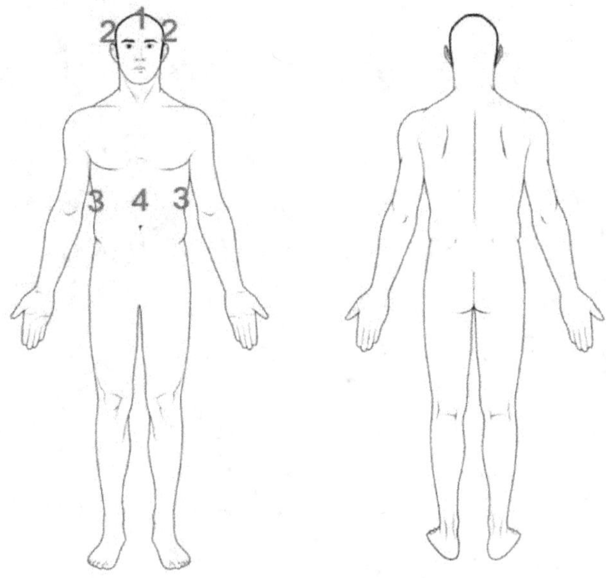

Accompanied symptom + Low fever

1. Hand placements: Head => chest and lung => chest and
hypochondrium .
2. Timing: 10'
3. Techniques: Cleansing + reducing + tonifying,
infiltrating methods

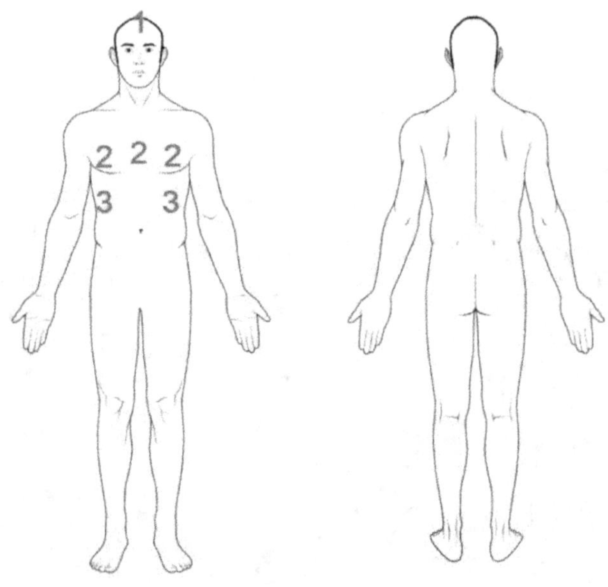

Accompanied symptom + headache

1. Hand placements: Back of head => overhead => lateral head => forehead
    a. wind-cold: + sides of neck
    b. wind-heat: + neck
    c. wind-dampness: + chest and hypochondrium
2. Timing: 10'
3. Techniques: Cleansing + reducing infiltrating methods

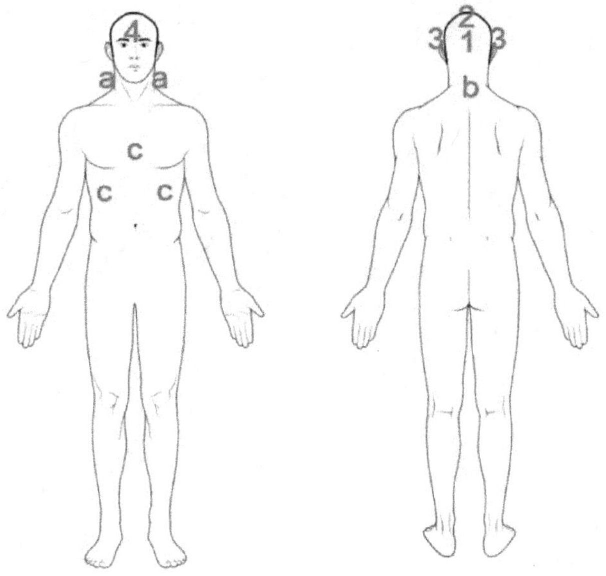

Accompanied symptom + immunity

1. Hand placements:
a. The front: lung => heart => chest and hypochondrium
b. The back: lung => heart => Kidneys
2. Timing: 10'
3. Techniques: Tonifying and infiltrating methods

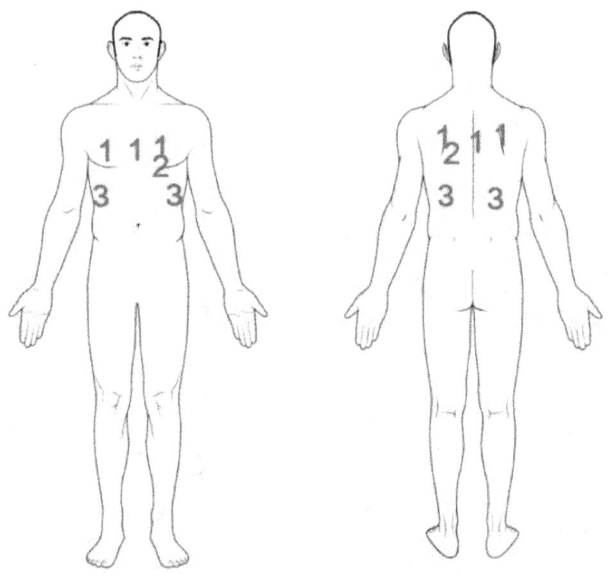

Your Healing Record #1

1. Hand placement:

2. Timing:

3. Techniques:

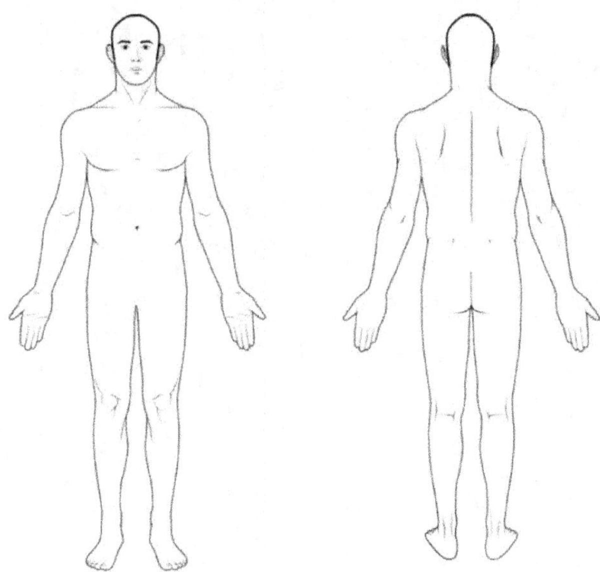

Your Healing Record #2

1. Hand placement:

2. Timing:

3. Techniques:

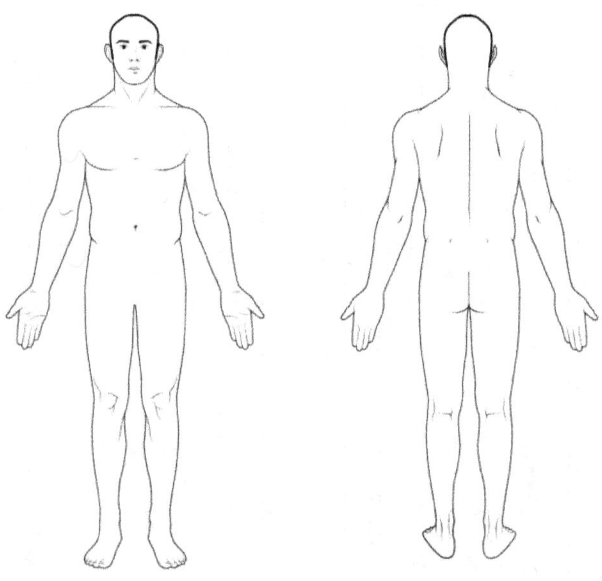

Abstain from :

1. Dairy
2. Strong tea, coffee, alcohol
3. Cold and raw food except mushrooms, garlic, ginger, and citrus fruits
4. Sugar, sweets
5. Seafood
6. Greasy and salty food

Nourishment

1. Sweet potato (containing vitamin A and L-Theanine)
2. Beef (containing zinc)
3. Yogurt (containing Lactobacillus reuteri)
4. Chicken soup (containing carnosine)
5. Mushroom (containing selenium)
6. Vitamin (B2, Niacin)
7. Garlic (rich in allicin)
8. Fresh ginger (anti-bacterial and anti-viral)
9. Fresh citrus (rich in vitamin C)

Nursing

1. Keep warm
2. Rest and sleep well.
3. Keep a light diet
4. Avoid crowds or confined space with many people
5. Wear a mask before going outdoors, cover with sleeves while coughing.
6. Wear a mask to avoid infection and warm up incoming air.

Warnings

Seek medical attention immediately if any of the following symptoms are present:

- Pain or pressure in the chest or abdomen
- Shortness of breath or difficulty breathing
- Skin color with a bluish or gray
- Green or bloody mucus
- Ear pain
- Lasting high fever
- Worsening asthma
- Seizure
- Sudden dizziness
- Mental confusion
- Severe or persistent vomiting